RENAL DIET SIDE DISHES AND APPETIZER COOKBOOK

Mouthwatering recipes to start renal diet.
The perfect renal food for your kidneys

Natalie Brown

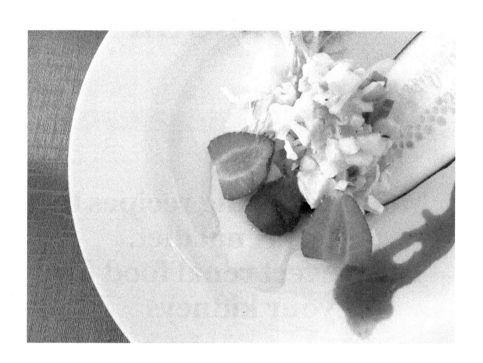

Table of Contents

As befitting its nature, it is presented without assurance regarding its prolonged validity or interim quality. Trademarks that are mentioned are done without written consent and can in no way be considered an endorsement from the trademark holder.

Introduction

Kidney disease is becoming more prevalent in the United States, and so we need to learn as much about it as we can. The more we educate ourselves, the more we can do to take care of this important bodily system. If you've been diagnosed with chronic kidney disease (CKD), education can empower you to most effectively and purposefully manage the disease. Once you have a full knowledge of what chronic kidney disease is, you can begin to take charge of your evolving health needs. Making healthy changes early in the stages of kidney disease will help determine how well you will manage your kidney health. I am here to guide you, every step of the way. Like any new process, it may seem intimidating at first.

What Do the Kidneys Do?

Our kidneys are small, but they do powerful things to keep our body in balance. They are bean-shaped, about the size of a fist, and are located in the middle of the back, on the left and right sides of the spine, just below the rib cage. When everything is working properly, the kidneys do many important jobs such as:

- Filter waste materials from the blood
- Remove extra fluid, or water, from the body
- Release hormones that help manage blood pressure
- Stimulate bone marrow to make red blood cells
- Make an active form of vitamin D that promotes strong, healthy bones

What Causes Kidney Disease?

There are many causes of kidney disease, including physical injury or disorders that can damage the kidneys, but the two leading causes of kidney disease are diabetes and high blood pressure. These underlying conditions also put people at risk for developing cardiovascular disease. Early treatment may not only slow down the progression of the disease, but also reduce your risk of developing heart disease or stroke.

Kidney disease can affect anyone, at any age. African Americans, Hispanics, and American Indians are at increased risk for kidney failure, because these groups have a greater prevalence of diabetes and high blood pressure.

When we digest Protein, our bodies create waste products. As blood flows through the capillaries, the waste products are filtered through the urine. Substances such as Protein and red blood cells are too big to pass through the capillaries and so stay in the blood. All the extra work takes a toll on the kidneys. When kidney disease is detected in the early stages, several treatments may prevent the worsening of the disease. If kidney disease is detected in the later stages, high amounts of Protein in your urine, called macro albuminuria, can lead to end-stage renal disease.

The second leading cause of kidney disease is high blood pressure, also known as hypertension. One in three Americans is at risk for kidney disease because of hypertension. Although there is no cure for hypertension, certain medications, a low-sodium diet, and physical activity can lower blood pressure.

The kidneys help manage blood pressure, but when blood pressure is high, the heart has to work overtime at pumping blood. When the force of blood flow is high, blood vessels start to stretch so the blood can flow more easily. The stretching and scarring weakens the blood vessels throughout the entire body, including the kidneys. And when the kidneys' blood vessels are injured, they may not remove the waste and extra fluid from the body, creating a dangerous cycle, because the extra fluid in the blood vessels can increase blood pressure even more.

With diabetes, excess blood sugar remains in the bloodstream. The high blood sugar levels can damage the blood vessels in the kidneys and elsewhere in the body. And since high blood pressure is a complication from diabetes, the extra pressure can weaken the walls of the blood vessels, which can lead to a heart attack or stroke.

Other conditions, such as drug abuse and certain autoimmune diseases, can also cause injury to the kidneys. In fact, every drug we put into our body has to pass through the kidneys for filtration.

An autoimmune disease is one in which the immune system, designed to protect the body from illness, sees the body as an invader and attacks its own systems, including the kidneys. Some forms of lupus, for example, attack the kidneys. Another autoimmune disease that can lead to kidney failure is Good pasture syndrome, a group of conditions that affect the kidneys and the lungs. The damage to the kidneys from autoimmune diseases can lead to chronic kidney disease and kidney failure.

Treatment Plans for Chronic Kidney Disease (CKD)

The best way to manage CKD is to be an active participant in your treatment program, regardless of your stage of renal disease. Proper treatment involves a combination of working with a healthcare team, adhering to a renal diet, and making healthy lifestyle decisions. These can all have a profoundly positive effect on your kidney disease—especially watching how you eat.

Working with your healthcare team. When you have kidney disease, working in partnership with your healthcare team can be extremely important in your treatment program as well as being personally empowering. Regularly meeting with your physician or healthcare team can arm you with resources and information that help you make informed decisions regarding your treatment needs, and provide you with a much needed opportunity to vent, share information, get advice, and receive support in effectively managing this illness.

Adhering to a renal diet. The heart of this book is the renal diet. Sticking to this diet can make a huge difference in your health and vitality. Like any change, following the diet may not be easy at first. Important changes to your diet, particularly early on, can possibly prevent the need for dialysis. These changes include limiting salt, eating a low-Protein diet, reducing Fat intake, and getting enough calories if you need to lose weight. Be honest with yourself first and foremost—learn what you need, and consider your personal goals and obstacles. Start by making small changes. It is okay to have some slip-ups—we all do. With guidance and support, these small changes will become habits of your promising new lifestyle. In no time, you will begin taking control of your diet and health.

Making healthy lifestyle decisions. Lifestyle choices play a crucial part in our health, especially when it comes to helping regulate kidney disease. Lifestyle choices such as allotting time for physical activity, getting enough sleep, managing weight, reducing stress, and limiting smoking and alcohol will help you take control of your overall health, making it easier to manage your kidney disease. Follow this simple formula: Keep toxins out of your body as much as you can, and build up your immune system with a good balance of exercise, relaxation, and sleep.

Stages of Kidney Disease

Based on the United States National Kidney Foundation, kidney disease can be classified into five different progressive stages. These stages and their symptoms do not only help the doctor to devise an appropriate therapy but also guide the patient to take the necessary measures in routine life. The rate of kidney function actually tells much about these phases. In the early stages, there is minimum loss of function, and this loss increases with every stage.

The eGFR is used as a standard criterion to measure the Kidney function. EGFR is the acronym for the estimated Glomerular Filtration Rate. It is the rate at which the waste material is transferred from the blood to the nephron's tubes through "glomerulus"- the filtering membrane of the kidney tissues. The lesser the rate of glomerular filtration, the greater the problem the kidneys are going through. A person's age, gender, race, and serum creatinine are entered into a mathematical formula to calculate his eGFR. The serum creatinine level is measured in a blood test. The creatinine is actually a waste product of the body which is produced out of muscular activities. Healthy kidneys are capable of removing all the creatinine out of the blood. A rising creatinine level is therefore a sign of kidney disease. It is said that if a person has been having an eGFR of less than 60 for three months, it means that he is suffering from serious renal problems.

There are five major stages of chronic kidney disease, and it can be categorized as follows:

Stage 1:

The first stage starts when the eGFR gets slightly higher than the normal value. In this stage, the eGFR can be equal or greater than 90mL/min

Stage 2:

The next stage arises when the eGFR starts to decline and ranges between 60 to 89 mL/min. It is best to control the progression of the disease at this point.

Stage 3:

From this point on, the kidney disease becomes concerning for the patient as the eGFR drops to 30-59 mL/min. At this stage, consultation is essential for the health of the patient.

Stage 4:

The stage 4 is also known as Severe Chronic Kidney Diseases as the eGFR level drops to 15-29 mL/min.

Stage 5:

The final and most critical phase of chronic renal disease is stage 5, where the estimated glomerular filtration rate gets as low as below 15 mL/min.

Role of Potassium, Sodium, and Phosphorus

1. Sodium

Sodium is considered the most important electrolyte of the body next to chloride and potassium. The electrolytes are actually the substance that controls the flow of fluids into the cells and out of them. Sodium is mainly responsible for regulating blood volume and pressure. It is also involved in controlling muscle contraction and nerve functions. The acid-base balance in the blood and other body fluids is also regulated by sodium. Though sodium is important for the health and regulation of important body mechanisms, excessive sodium intake, especially when a person suffers from some stages of chronic kidney disease, can be dangerous. Excess sodium disrupts the critical fluid balance in the body and inside the kidneys. It then leads to high blood pressure, which in turn negatively affects the kidneys. Salt is one of the major sources of sodium in our diet, and it is strictly forbidden on the renal diet. High sodium intake can also lead to Edema, which is swelling of the face, hands, and legs. Furthermore, high blood pressure can stress the heart and cause the weakening of its muscles. The build-up of fluid in the lungs also leads to shortness of breath.

2. Potassium

Potassium is another mineral that is closely linked to renal health. Potassium is another important electrolyte, so it maintains the fluid balance in the body and its pH levels as well. This electrolyte also plays a vital role in controlling nerve impulses and muscular activity. It works in conjugation with the sodium to carry out all these functions. The normal potassium level in the blood must range between 3.5 and 5.5mEq/L. It is the kidneys that help maintain this balance, but without their proper function, the potassium starts to build up in the blood. Hyperkalemia is a condition characterized by high potassium levels. It usually occurs in people with chronic kidney disease. The prominent symptoms of high potassium are numbness, slow pulse rate, weakness, and nausea. Potassium is present in green vegetables and some fruits, and these ingredients should be avoided on a renal diet.

3. Phosphorus

The amount of phosphorus in the blood is largely linked to the functioning of the kidneys. Phosphorus, in combination with vitamin D, calcium, and parathyroid hormone, can regulate the renal function. The balance of phosphorous and calcium is maintained by the kidneys, and this balance keeps the bones and teeth healthy. Phosphorus, along with vitamin D, ensures the absorption of calcium into the bones and teeth, where this mineral is important for the body. On the other hand, it gets dangerous when the kidneys fail to control the amount of phosphorus in the blood. This may lead to heart and bone-related problems. Mainly there is a high risk of weakening of the bones followed by the hardening of the tissues due to the deposition of phosphorous and calcium outside the bones. This abnormal calcification can occur in the lungs, skin, joints, and arteries, which can become in time very painful. It may also result in bone pain and itching.

What is Renal Diet?

A renal diet is an eating plan exercised to help minimize waste products' levels in the blood. The renal diet is designed to cause as little work or stress on the kidneys as possible, while still providing energy and the high nutrients the body needs.

A renal diet follows several fundamental guidelines. The first is that it must be a balanced, healthy, and sustainable diet, rich in natural grains, vitamins, fibers, carbohydrates, omega 3 fats, and fluids. Proteins should be adequate, but not excessive.

Accumulates in the blood are kept to a minimum. Blood electrolyte levels are monitored regularly, and the diet corrected. It is essential to follow specific advice from your doctor and dietitian.

Daily Protein intake is essential to rebuild tissues but needs to be kept to a minimum. Superfluous proteins need to be broken down by the body into nitrates and carbs. Nitrates are not employed by the body and have to be excreted via the kidneys.

Carbs are an important source of energy and should be taken in adequate amounts. Whole grains are the best. Avoid highly refined carbohydrates.

Table salt ought to be limited to cooking only. Excess salt overworks the kidneys and causes fluid retention. Salty foods like processed meats, lots of foods, sausages, and snacks should be avoided.

Phosphorus is essential for the body to function, but dialysis can't remove it, so amounts need to be monitored, and intake should be restricted though not eliminated completely.

Foods, like dairy products, darker drinks such as colas and legumes, have high phosphorus content. If levels of this increase in the blood, foods high in potassium such as citrus fruits and dark, leafy green lettuce, carrots or apricots might have to be restricted.

Omega 3 fats are a significant part of any healthy diet. Fish is an excellent source. Omega fats are important for the body. Avoid trans-fats or hydrolyzed fats.

Fluids should be enough but might need to be limited in cases of fluid retention.

A healthy renal diet can help keep kidney function for longer. The main differences between a renal diet and any nutritious diet plan are the limitations placed on Protein and table salt ingestion. Restrictions on fluids and potassium might become necessary as signs and symptoms of accumulation become evident.

For people with diabetes who also suffer from kidney disease, there is a food strategy or diet. Over fifty percent of chronic kidney disease sufferers are people that have diabetes, indicating the necessity for them to stick to the diabetic diet.

In several cases, this diet is prepared and is effective in different phases of this disease. There are also instances where the diet is created for people with diabetes hoping to avoid renal disorder. Sufferers of diabetes and kidney problems have trouble eating the proper food.

The aim of a diabetic's meal plan would be to get the blood within the safe selection. This may be carried out just by having meals frequently on a daily basis, not missing any, and eating carbohydrate foods that are low glycemic.

Consuming a number of such carbohydrates at every meal can assist the body in maintaining a moderate blood sugar level, becoming neither too high nor too low.

Low glycemic foods include brown rice, sweet potatoes, and whole-grain bread. But if it is a renal diet for diabetics, whole-grain bread and sweet potatoes ought not to be used since they're rich in potassium.

For people with kidney issues, they should eat less of these foods full of potassium, phosphorus and sodium. A blood sugar-lowering diet for people with diabetes can be a diet suitable for renal issues. Patients need to check labels since sodium is common in several foods.

For clients with kidney problems, dietitians advice against the consumption of diet pops of java because such drinks contain sodium.

On a diabetic-renal meal plan, unsweetened teas, water and diet sodas are allowed. When it comes to vegetables, broccoli, cauliflower, beets, eggplant, and cabbage are usually recommended because of their abundant vitamin content and very low carbohydrate and potassium content. Meats that are rich in sodium, such as organ meats, sausage, and bacon, ought not to be taken.

Since canned vegetables contain lots of sodium, it is necessary to choose raw vegetables and steer clear of the canned variety. Furthermore, raw vegetables are more nutritious, considering their vitamins.

It is recommended that people with diabetes learn from certified nutritionists the foods that they need to eat or avoid.

However, all forms of renal diet have one thing in common, which is to improve your renal functions, bring some relief to your kidneys, as well as prevent kidneys disease at patients with numerous risk factors, altogether improving your overall health and wellbeing. The grocery list we have provided should help you get ahold of which groceries you should introduce to your diet and which groups of food should be avoided in order to improve your kidneys' performance, so you can start from shopping for your new lifestyle.

You don't need to shop many different types of groceries all at once as it is always better to use fresh produce, although frozen food also makes a good alternative when fresh fruit and vegetables are not available.

As far as the renal diet we are recommending in our guide, this form of kidney-friendly dietary regimen offer solution in form of low-sodium and low-potassium meals and groceries, which is why we are also offering simple and easy renal diet recipes in our guide. By following a dietary plan compiled for all stages of renal system failure unless the doctor recommends a different treatment by allowing or expelling some of the groceries, we have listed in our ultimate grocery list for renal patients.

Before we get to cooking and changing your lifestyle from the very core with the idea of improving your health, we want you to get familiar with renal diet basics and find out exactly what his diet is based on while you already know what is the very core solution found in renal diet – helping you improve your kidney's health by lowering sodium and potassium intake.

The best way of getting familiar with renal diet and basics of this dietary regimen is to take a look at the most commonly asked questions that extend the answer to a question what is renal diet?

Benefits of Renal Diet

If you have been diagnosed with kidney dysfunction, a proper diet is necessary for controlling the amount of toxic waste in the bloodstream. When toxic waste piles up in the system along with increased fluid, chronic inflammation occurs and we have a much higher chance of developing cardiovascular, bone, metabolic or other health issues.

Since your kidneys can't fully get rid of waste on their own, which comes from food and drinks, probably the only natural way to help our system is through this diet.

A renal diet is especially useful during the first stages of kidney dysfunction and leads to the following benefits:

Prevents excess fluid and waste build-up

Prevents the progression of renal dysfunction stages

Decreases the likelihood of developing other chronic health problems e.g. heart disorders

Has a mild antioxidant function in the body, which keeps inflammation and inflammatory responses under control.

The above mentioned benefits are noticeable once the patient follows the diet for at least a month and then continuing it for longer periods, to avoid the stage where dialysis is needed. The strictness of the diet depends on the current stage of renal/kidney disease, if, for example, you are in the 3rd or 4th stage, you should follow a stricter diet and be attentive for the food, which is allowed or prohibited.

These exact foods and nutrients that you should take when following a renal diet, will be given to you in the following sections, and so keep on reading.

Explanation of key diet words

The following nutrients play a major role in a renal diet as some have the ability to improve the condition while others can make it worse. Essentially, renal diet is based on low consumption of certain nutrients like potassium and phosphorus simply because it promotes fluid buildup within the system of a kidney patient. Here is a brief explanation of the function of each nutrient and its role in a renal diet:

Potassium.

Potassium is a mineral that naturally occurs in certain foods and plays a role in regulating heart rhythm and muscle movement. It is also needed for keeping fluid and electrolyte balance in normal levels. Our kidneys keep only the right levels of potassium in our system, and when it is excess, they expel it via the urine.

The problem is, once kidneys can't function properly, all this excess potassium can't be expelled out and spikes up, causing symptoms like muscle and bone weakness, abnormal heartbeat, and heart failure in extreme cases.

Thus, a diet low in potassium is recommended to prevent buildup and avoid such negative side effects.

Sodium.

Sodium is a trace mineral that is found in most foods that we eat today and it is the key component of salt, which is actually a sodium compound mixed with chloride. Most food that we consume and especially processed food is highly loaded with salt, however, we may be eating sodium in other forms too e.g. fish. The key role of sodium is to regulate blood pressure, help regulate nerve function, and maintain the balance of acids in the blood. However, when sodium is excessively high and the kidneys can expel it, it can lead to the following symptoms: an elevated feeling of thirst, swelling of hands, feet and the face, elevated blood pressure, and problems with breathing.

This is why it is suggested to keep sodium intake low, to avoid the above.

Phosphorus.

Phosphorus is an essential mineral that is responsible for the development and regeneration of our bones. Phosphorus also plays a key role in the growth of connective tissue e.g. muscles and the regulation of muscle motions. When food we take contains phosphorus, it gets absorbed by the intestines and then gets deposited in our bones.

However, when kidneys are damaged or dysfunctioning, the excess phosphorus can't be expelled through our systems and causes problems such as: extracting calcium out of the bones/making them weaker, and leading to excess calcium in the bloodstream which interferes with blood vessels, heart, eye, and lung function.

Protein.

Protein is a nutritional compound that consists of amino acids, which play a key role in various system functions like cell communication, oxygen supply, and cellular metabolism. They are also a part of a healthy immune system.

Normally, Protein is not an issue for our kidneys. When Protein is metabolized, waste by-products are also created and are filtered through the kidneys. This waste along with extra renal proteins after will be expelled through urine.

However, when kidneys are unable to filter out excess Protein, it gets accumulated in the blood and cause problems.

This doesn't mean that renal disease patients should avoid Protein totally as it is still necessary for some metabolic functions, as long as it's taken in moderate amounts and based on the stage of renal disease.

Carbs.

Carbs act as a key source of fuel for our bodies. The consumption of carbs is turned into glucose in our system, which is a primary source of energy.

Carbs are ok to be eaten in moderation by kidney patients and the daily recommended allowance is up to 150 grams/day. However, patients that also have Diabetes (besides renal disease) should control their carb consumption to avoid any sudden spikes in their blood glucose.

Fat.

Being in balanced amounts, fats in our bodies act as an energy source, aid in the release of hormones, and help regulate blood pressure. They also carry some vitamins that are Fat-soluble such as A, D, E, and K, which are also very important for our systems. Not all fats are created equal still, few are good for our health and some are bad. Bad fats are saturated and Trans fats and are found in processed meat, dairy, and other products. They are also found in margarine and vegetable Fat shortenings.

Fat, in general, don't pose a risk for renal disease patients, however, it is suggested to limit the consumption of saturated and Tran's fats to avoid any cardiovascular problems e.g. elevated blood pressure and clogging of the arteries.

Dietary Fiber.

Dietary Fiber is a compound that can't be digested on its own by enzymes and acids in our stomach and intestines, but is needed for the system to aid in the digestion of our food and encourage bowel movements. They generally promote bowel regularity and decrease the likelihood of developing constipation inside the colon. Dietary Fiber is typically found in fruits, vegetables, seeds and whole grains.

In patients with renal disease, dietary Fiber is ok up to 28 grams/day as long as these plant foods don't contain high amounts of phosphorus or potassium.

Vitamins.

According to medical and dietary guidelines, our bodies need close to 13 vitamins to functions. Vitamins play a key role in metabolic functions and the normal functioning of our cardiovascular, digestive, nervous system and immune systems. The adoption of a nutritionally dense and balanced diet is necessary for getting all the vitamins our system needs. However, due to some diet restrictions e.g. sodium, many renal patients are in need of water-soluble vitamins like B-complex (B1, B2, B6, B12, folic acid, biotin) and small amounts of Vitamin C.

Minerals.

Minerals are needed for our system to maintain healthy connective tissue e.g. bones, muscles, and skin and facilitate the normal function of our hearts and central nervous systems.

Our kidneys typically expel any excess amount of minerals through our urine as some can lead to health symptoms e.g. muscle spasms when their levels are abnormally high.

However, as it was mentioned earlier, some minerals like potassium and phosphorus cannot be expelled by our kidneys when in excess and so their intake through diet should be limited.

Other trace minerals are perfectly fine when following a renal diet: iron, copper, zinc and selenium. A lack of these can lead to increased oxidative stress and thus, it is important to take sufficient amounts through diet or supplementation.

Fluids.

Fluids are necessary for the proper hydration of our systems in fact; lack of fluids can lead to dehydration and death in extreme cases.

However, in patients with renal dysfunction, fluids can quickly build up to the point of placing pressure to vital organs like the lungs and heart and becoming dangerous. This is the reason why many physicians advise their kidney patients to limit the consumption of fluids, especially during the last stages of the disorder.

Managing Kidney Disease through Diet

Patients who struggle from kidney health issues, going through kidney dialysis and have renal impairments need to not only go through medical treatment but also change their eating habit, lifestyle to make the situation better. Numerous researches have been finished on this, and the conclusion is food has a lot to do with how your kidney functions and its overall health.

The first thing to changing your lifestyle is knowing about how your kidney functions and how different food can trigger different reactions in the kidney function. There are certain nutrients that affect your kidney directly. Nutrients like sodium, Protein, phosphate, and potassium are the risky ones. You do not have to omit them altogether from your diet, but you need to limit or minimize their intake as much as possible. You cannot leave out essential nutrient like Protein from your diet, but you need to count how much Protein you are having per day. This is essential in order to keep balance in your muscles and maintaining a good functioning kidney.

A vast change in kidney patients is measuring how much fluid they are drinking. This is a crucial change in every kidney patient, and you must adapt to this new eating habit. Too much water or any other form of liquid can disrupt your kidney function. How much fluid you can consume depends on the condition of your kidney. Most people assign separate bottles for them so that they can measure how much they have drunk and how much more they can drink throughout the day.

What You Can and Can't Eat

Food to Eat

The renal diet aims to cut down the amount of waste in the blood. When people have kidney dysfunction, the kidneys are unable to remove and filter waste properly. When waste is left in the blood, it can affect the electrolyte levels of the patient. With a kidney diet, kidney function is promoted, and the progression of complete kidney failure is slowed down.

The renal diet follows a low intake of Protein, phosphorus, and sodium. It is necessary to consume high-quality Protein and limit some fluids. For some people, it is important to limit calcium and potassium.

Promoting a renal diet, here are the substances which are critical to be monitored:

Sodium and its role in the body

Most natural foods contain sodium. Some people think that sodium and salt are interchangeable. However, salt is a compound of chloride and sodium. There might be either salt or sodium in other forms in the food we eat. Due to the added salt, processed foods include a higher level of sodium.

Apart from potassium and chloride, sodium is one of the most crucial body's electrolytes. The main function of electrolytes is to control the fluids when they are going out and in the body's cells and tissues.

With sodium:

Blood volume and pressure are regulated.

Muscle contraction and nerve function are regulated.

The acid-base balance of the blood is regulated.

The amount of fluid the body eliminates and keeps is balanced.

Why is it important to monitor sodium intake for people with kidney issues?

Since the kidneys of kidney disease patients are unable to reduce excess fluid and sodium from the body adequately, too much sodium might be harmful. As fluid and sodium build up in the bloodstream and tissues, they might cause:

Edema: swelling in face, hands, and legs

Increased thirst

High blood pressure

Shortness of breath

Heart failure

The ways to monitor sodium intake:

Avoid processed foods

Be attentive to serving sizes.

Read food labels

Utilize fresh meats instead of processed

Choose fresh fruits and veggies.

Compare brands, choosing the ones with the lowest sodium levels.

Utilize spices that do not include salt

Ensure the sodium content is less than 400 mg per meal and not more than 150 mg per snack

Cook at home, not adding salt

Foods to eat with lower sodium content:

Fresh meats, dairy products, frozen veggies, and fruits

Fresh herbs and seasonings like rosemary, oregano, dill, lime, cilantro, onion, lemon, and garlic

Corn tortilla chips, pretzels, no salt added crackers, unsalted popcorn

Potassium and its role in the body

The main function of potassium is keeping muscles working correctly and the heartbeat regular. This mineral is responsible for maintaining electrolyte and fluid balance in the bloodstream. The kidneys regulate the proper amount of potassium in the body, expelling excess amounts in the urine.

Monitoring potassium intake

Limit high potassium food

Select only fresh fruits and veggies

Limit dairy products and milk to 8 oz. per day

Avoid potassium chloride

Read labels on packaged foods.

Avoid seasonings and salt substitutes with potassium.

Foods to eat with lower potassium:

Fruits: watermelon, tangerines, pineapple, plums, peaches, pears, papayas, mangoes, lemons and limes, honeydew, grapefruit/grapefruit juice, grapes/grape juice, clementine/satsuma, cranberry juice, berries, and apples/ applesauce, apple juice

Veggies: summer squash (cooked), okra, mushrooms (fresh), lettuce, kale, green beans, eggplant, cucumber, corn, onions (raw), celery, cauliflower, carrots, cabbage, broccoli (fresh), bamboo shoots (canned), and bell peppers

Plain Turkish delights, marshmallows and jellies, boiled fruit sweets, and peppermints

Shortbread, ginger nut biscuits, plain digestives

Plain flapjacks and cereal bars

Plain sponge cakes like Madeira cake, lemon sponge, jam sponge

Corn-based and wheat crisps

Whole grain crispbreads and crackers

Protein and other foods (bread (not whole grain), pasta, noodles, rice, eggs, canned tuna, turkey (white meat), and chicken (white meat)

Phosphorus and its role in the body

This mineral is essential in bone development and maintenance. Phosphorus helps in the development of connective organs and tissue and assists in muscle movement. Extra phosphorus is possible to be removed by healthy kidneys. However, it is impossible with kidney dysfunction. High levels of phosphorus make bones weak by pulling calcium out of your bones. It might lead to dangerous calcium deposits in the heart, eyes, lungs, and blood vessels.

Monitoring phosphorus intake

Pay attention to serving size

Eat fresh fruits and veggies

Eat smaller portions of foods that are rich in Protein

Avoid packaged foods

Keep a food journal

Foods to eat with low phosphorus level:

Grapes, apples

Lettuce, leeks

Carbs (white rice, corn, and rice Cereal, popcorn, pasta, crackers (not wheat), white bread)

Meat (sausage, fresh meat)

Protein

Damaged kidneys are unable to remove Protein waste, so they accumulate in the blood. The amount of Protein to consume differs depending on the stage of CKD. Protein is critical for tissue maintenance, and it is necessary to eat the proper amount of it according to the particular stage of kidneys disease.

Sources of Protein for vegetarians:

Vegans (allowing only plant-based foods): Wheat Protein and whole grains, nut butter, soy Protein, yogurt or soy milk, cooked no salt added canned and dried beans and peas, unsalted nuts.

Lacto vegetarians (allowing dairy products, milk, and plant-based foods): reduced-sodium or low-sodium cottage cheese.

Lacto-Ovo vegetarians (allowing eggs, dairy products, milk, and plant-based foods): eggs.

Food to Avoid

Food with high sodium content:

Onion salt, marinades, garlic salt, teriyaki sauce, and table salt

Pepperoni, bacon, ham, lunch meat, hot dogs, sausage, processed meats

Ramen noodles, canned produce, and canned soups

Marinara sauce, gravy, salad dressings, soy sauce, BBQ sauce, and ketchup

Chex Mix, salted nuts, Cheetos, crackers, and potato chips

Fast food

Food with a high potassium level:

Fruits: dried fruit, oranges/orange juice, prunes/prune juice, kiwi, nectarines, dates, cantaloupe, bananas, black currants, damsons, cherries, grapes, and apricots.

Vegetables: tomatoes/tomato sauce/tomato juice, sweet potatoes, beans, lentils, split peas, spinach (cooked), pumpkin, potatoes, mushrooms (cooked), chile peppers, chard, Brussels sprouts (cooked), broccoli (cooked), baked beans, avocado, butternut squash, and acorn squash.

Protein and other foods: peanut butter, molasses, granola, chocolate, bran, sardines, fish, bacon, ham, nuts and seeds, yogurt, milkshakes, and milk.

Coconut-based snacks, nut-based snacks, fudge, and toffee

Cakes containing marzipan.

Potato crisps.

Foods with high phosphorus:

Dairy products: pudding, ice cream, yogurt, cottage cheese, cheese, and milk

Nuts and seeds: sunflower seeds, pumpkin seeds, pecans, peanut butter, pistachios, cashews, and almonds

Dried beans and peas: soybeans, split peas, refried beans, pinto beans, lentils, kidney beans, garbanzo beans, black beans, and baked beans.

Meat: veal, turkey, liver, lamb, beef, bacon, fish, and seafood.

Carbs: whole grain products, oatmeal, and bran cereals

Chapter 1. Renal Diet Side Dishes and Appetizer Recipes

1. Popcorn with Sugar and Spice

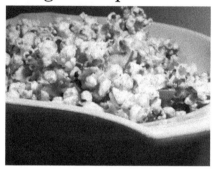

Preparation Time: 5 minutes

Cooking Time: 10 minutes

Servings: 3

Ingredients:

- 8 cups hot popcorn
- 2 tablespoons unsalted butter
- 2 tablespoons sugar
- 1/2 teaspoon cinnamon
- 1/4 teaspoon nutmeg

Directions:

1. Popping the corn; put aside.

2. Heat the butter, sugar, cinnamon, and nutmeg in the microwave or saucepan over a range fire until the butter is melted and the sugar dissolved.

3. Be careful not to burn the butter.

4. Sprinkle the corn with the spicy butter, mix well.

5. Serve immediately for optimal flavor.

Nutrition:

Calories: 120 kcal

Total Fat: 7 g

Saturated Fat: 0 g

Cholesterol: 16 mg

Sodium: 2 mg

Total Carbs: 12 g

Fiber: 2.5 g

Sugar: 0 g

Phosphorus 4 mg

Potassium 9 mg

Protein: 2 g

2. Baked Pita Chips

Preparation Time: 5 minutes

Cooking Time: 15 minutes

Servings: 6

Ingredients:

- 3 pita loaves (6 inches)
- 3 tablespoons olive oil
- Chili powder

Directions:

1. Separate each bread in half with scissors, to obtain 6 round pieces. Cut each piece into eight points. Brush each with olive oil and sprinkle with chili powder. Bake at 350 degrees F for about 15 minutes until crisp.

Nutrition:

Calories: 120 kcal

Total Fat: 2.5 g

Saturated Fat: 0 g

Cholesterol: 0 mg

Sodium: 70 mg

Total Carbs: 22 g

Fiber: 1 g

Sugar: 0 g

Protein: 3 g

Phosphorus 25 mg

Potassium 24 mg

3. Energy Bars

Preparation Time: 10 minutes

Cooking Time: 40 minutes

Servings: 8

Ingredients:

- .5 tsp. of ground cinnamon
- .25 cup of semi-sweet chocolate chips
- 9 tsp. of chopped up unsalted peanuts
- 8 oz. of rolled oats
- .33 cup of shredded coconut
- .33 cup of applesauce
- 3 eggs (large)
- 9 tsp. of honey

Directions:

1. Heat to 325 and grease a 9x9 pan.

2. Combine rolled oats, cinnamon, peanuts, coconut, and chocolate chips together.

3. Beat together the eggs, applesauce, and honey. Mix well.

4. Combine together oats and eggs. Make sure to mix thoroughly.

5. Place mixture into pan that was previously prepared and pat down. Cook for forty minutes. Allow to cool & then cut into bars. Will keep for seven days refrigerated in a sealed container.

Nutrition:

Calories: 206 kcal

Total Fat: 0 g

Saturated Fat: 0 g

Cholesterol: 0 mg

Sodium: 35 mg

Total Carbs: 27 g

Fiber: 0 g

Sugar: 0 g

Protein: 7 g

Phosphorus 256 mg

Potassium 238 mg

4. Strawberry Gelatin Power Cubes (High Protein)

Preparation Time: 10 minutes

Cooking Time: 30 minutes

Servings: 8

Ingredients:

- 2 cups of water
- 1 box of original unflavored gelatin (four envelopes)
- cups of cold water
- 3 boxes gelatin (strawberry, sugar-free)
- 1 and 2/3 cups of strawberry flavored whey Protein

Directions:

1. Bring the 2 cups water to a boil (either microwave or on the stovetop).

2. Slowly add the strawberry gelatin and stir until completely dissolved.

3. Using a shaking container, pour in the water (cold), unflavored gelatin, plus the whey Protein. Combine so that the contents are smooth without chunks.

4. Introduce the whey Protein to the strawberry gelatin and continuously stir.

5. Evacuate mixture from bowl to the 9x13 pan. Cover and chill until the mixture becomes firm. Cut into forty-eight pieces.

Nutrition:

Calories: 80 kcal

Total Fat: 0 g

Saturated Fat: 0 g

Cholesterol: 0 mg

Sodium: 74 mg

Total Carbs: 3 g

Fiber: 0 g

Sugar: 0 g

Protein: 17 g

Phosphorus 160 mg

Potassium 61 mg

5. Pb & J Celery Sticks

Preparation Time: 5 minutes

Cooking Time: 0 minute

Servings: 4

Ingredients:

- 4 tablespoons of creamy peanut butter
- 6 tsp. of jelly
- 4 celery stalks (medium-sized, around 8 inches)

Directions:

1. Trim up the celery and rinse.

2. Fill each one using 1 tsp. peanut spread and one-fourth jelly.

3. Cut each of the stalks into three pieces and serve.

Nutrition:

Calories: 90 kcal

Total Fat: 8 g

Saturated Fat: 0 g

Cholesterol: 0 mg

Sodium: 103 mg

Total Carbs: 12 g

Fiber: 1 g

Sugar: 0 g

Protein: 4 g

Phosphorus 24 mg

Potassium 93 mg

6. Spanish rice

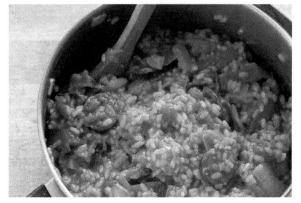

Preparation Time: 5 minutes

Cooking Time: 20 minutes

Servings: 2

Ingredients:

- White rice – .75 cup
- Chicken broth, low sodium– 1.5 cups
- Onion dehydrated flakes – 2 tablespoons
- Garlic, minced – 2 cloves
- Lemon juice – 1 tablespoon
- Cumin, ground - .25 teaspoon
- Chili powder - .5 teaspoon
- Oregano, dried - .5 teaspoon
- Black pepper, ground - .25 teaspoon
- Cilantro, chopped – 3 tablespoons

Directions:

1. Unlike most Spanish rice, this one does not contain tomatoes. However, it is still high on flavors and you will find it is the

perfect addition for tacos, burritos, and simply as a side dish whenever you crave a burst of flavor.

2. Place the rice, chicken broth, onion flakes, and minced garlic in a medium-sized saucepan. Bring the chicken broth and rice to a boil over medium heat, and then reduce the heat to a light simmer, cover it with a lid, and allow it to cook until the liquid has all been absorbed about eighteen to twenty minutes.

3. Use a fork to fluff the rice mix in the lemon juice, cumin, chili powder, oregano, black pepper, and cilantro. Once combined, serve the rice while still warm.

Nutrition:

Calories: 303 kcal

Total Fat: 1 g

Saturated Fat: 0 g

Cholesterol: 0 mg

Sodium: 57 mg

Total Carbs: 65 g

Fiber: 0 g

Sugar: 0 g

Protein: 6 g

Phosphorus 73 mg

Potassium 176 mg

7. Mushroom Orzo

Preparation Time: 5 minutes

Cooking Time: 20 minutes

Servings: 2

Ingredients:

- Orzo - .75 cup
- Chicken broth, low-sodium – 1.25 cup
- Mushrooms, diced – 4 ounces
- Garlic, minced – 3 cloves
- Onion flakes, dehydrated – 1 tablespoon
- Olive oil – 1 tablespoon
- Sage, ground - .25 teaspoon

Directions:

1. Orzo is a type of pasta formed in the shape of rice. It has a wonderful flavor and texture, and due to the small sizes, it greatly absorbs the flavor of whatever it is cooked. You will love this orzo with the addition of mushrooms, garlic, and sage.

2. Place the diced mushrooms, olive oil, and garlic in a medium-sized metal saucepan and allow them to sauté over medium heat for five minutes. Add in the sage, onion flakes, orzo, and low-sodium chicken broth. Bring the mixture to a boil.

3. Reduce the heat of the skillet to a light simmer, cover the pot with a lid, and allow it to cook until all of the liquid has been absorbed about nine minutes. Fluff the orzo with a fork before serving.

Nutrition:

Calories: 337 kcal

Total Fat: 8 g

Saturated Fat: 0 g

Cholesterol: 0 mg

Sodium: 43 mg

Total Carbs: 99 g

Fiber: 0 g

Sugar: 0 g

Protein: 18 g

Phosphorus 59 mg

Potassium 181 mg

8. Carrot and Pineapple Slaw

Preparation Time: 5 minutes

Cooking Time: 0 minute

Servings: 2

Ingredients:

- Carrot matchsticks – 5 ounces
- Pineapple chunks, canned, liquid drained - .5 cup
- Grapes, sliced in half - .5 cup
- Pecan pieces - .25 cup
- Mayonnaise, low-sodium - .33 cup
- Lemon juice – 1 tablespoon

Directions:

1. This slaw is sweet and savory with the pineapple and grapes perfectly complementing the carrots. You will especially love that this slaw can be made up to a day in advance, making it the perfect side dish to take with you to work, on a road trip, or to a potluck.

2. In a bowl, toss together the carrot matchsticks, drained pineapple chunks, sliced grapes, and pecan pieces. Stir in the low-sodium mayonnaise and lemon juice.

3. Cover the bowl with plastic wrap or a lid and then allow it to chill and marinate for at least an hour before serving. You can make this slaw up to a day in advance.

Nutrition:

Calories: 264 kcal

Total Fat: 17 g

Saturated Fat: 0 g

Cholesterol: 0 mg

Sodium: 91 mg

Total Carbs: 29 g

Fiber: 0 g

Sugar: 0 g

Protein: 2 g

Phosphorus 62 mg

Potassium 409 mg

9. Cucumber Salad

Preparation Time: 5 minutes

Cooking Time: 5 minutes

Servings: 4

Ingredients:

- 1 tbsp. dried dill
- 1 onion
- 1/4 cup water
- 1 cup vinegar
- 3 cucumbers
- 3/4 cup white sugar

Directions:

1. In a bowl add ingredients and mix well

2. Serve with dressing

Nutrition:

Calories: 49 kcal

Total Fat: 0.1 g

Saturated Fat: 0 g

Cholesterol: 0 mg

Sodium: 341 mg

Total Carbs: 11 g

Fiber: 0 g

Sugar: 0 g

Protein: 0.8 g

Phosphorus 49 mg

Potassium 309 mg

10. Thai Cucumber Salad

Preparation Time: 5 minutes

Cooking Time: 5 minutes

Servings: 2

Ingredients:

- 1/4 cup chopped peanuts
- 1/4 cup white sugar
- 1/2 cup cilantro
- 1/4 cup rice wine vinegar
- 3 cucumbers
- 2 jalapeno peppers

Directions:

1. In a bowl add ingredients and mix well

2. Serve with dressing

Nutrition:

Calories: 20 kcal

Total Fat: 0 g

Saturated Fat: 0 g

Cholesterol: 0 mg

Sodium: 85 mg

Total Carbs: 5 g

Fiber: 0 g

Sugar: 0 g

Protein: 1 g

Phosphorus 204 mg

Potassium 718 mg

11. Red Potato Salad

Preparation Time: 5 minutes

Cooking Time: 5 minutes

Servings: 2

Ingredients:

- 2 cups mayonnaise
- 1 lb. bacon
- 1 stalk celery
- 4 eggs
- Pepper.
- 2 lbs. red potatoes
- 1 onion

Directions:

1. In a pot add water, potatoes and cook until tender

2. Remove, drain and set aside

3. Place eggs in a saucepan, add water and bring to a boil

4. Cover and let eggs stand for 10-15 minutes

5. When ready remove, meanwhile in a deep skillet cook bacon on low heat

6. In a bowl add ingredients and mix well

7. Serve with dressing

Nutrition:

Calories: 280 kcal

Total Fat: 20 g

Saturated Fat: 0 g

Cholesterol: 0 mg

Sodium: 180 mg

Total Carbs: 26 g

Fiber: 0 g

Sugar: 0 g

Protein: 2 g

Phosphorus 889 mg

Potassium 3098 mg

12. Rosemary and Roasted Cauliflower

Preparation Time: 10 minutes

Cooking Time: 30 minutes

Servings: 1

Ingredients:

- 11/2 tablespoons olive oil
- 1 medium head cauliflower
- 1/4 teaspoon salt
- 1 tablespoon fresh rosemary, finely chopped
- Fresh ground black pepper

Directions:

1. Heat up an oven to 450°F.

2. Cut florets from cauliflower head. Cut into bite-size pieces.

3. Toss the cauliflower w/ the rest of the ingredients in a large bowl.

4. Spread the seasoned cauliflower on an ungreased baking sheet.

5. Roast for 15 minutes. Remove from oven and stir.

6. Cook for 10 minutes until the cauliflower is tender.

Nutrition:

Protein - 1g;

Phosphorus: 23mg;

Potassium: 124mg;

Sodium: 27mg;

Carbs - 2g;

Fat - 2g;

Calories – 32.

13. Broccoli-Cauliflower Salad

Preparation Time: 5 minutes

Cooking Time: 5 minutes

Servings: 4

Ingredients:

- 1 tbsp. wine vinegar
- 1 cup cauliflower florets
- 1/4 cup white sugar
- 2 cups hard-cooked eggs
- 5 slices bacon
- 1 cup broccoli florets
- 1 cup cheddar cheese
- 1 cup mayonnaise

Directions:

1. In a bowl add ingredients and mix well

2. Serve with dressing

Nutrition:

Calories: 89.8 kcal

Total Fat: 4.5 g

Saturated Fat: 0 g

Cholesterol: 0 mg

Sodium: 51.2 mg

Total Carbs: 11.5 g

Fiber: 0 g

Sugar: 0 g

Phosphorus 224 mg

Potassium 391 mg

Protein: 3 g

14. Macaroni Salad

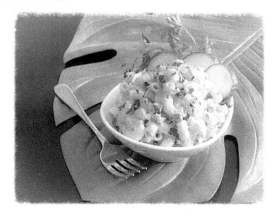

Preparation Time: 5 minutes

Cooking Time: 5 minutes

Servings: 4

Ingredients:

- 1/4 tsp. celery seed
- 2 hard-boiled eggs
- 2 cups salad dressing
- 1 onion
- 2 tsps. white vinegar
- 2 stalks celery
- 2 cups cooked macaroni
- 1 red bell pepper
- 2 tbsps. mustard

Directions:

1. In a bowl add ingredients and mix well

2. Serve with dressing

Nutrition:

Calories: 360 kcal

Total Fat: 21 g

Saturated Fat: 0 g

Cholesterol: 0 mg

Sodium: 400 mg

Total Carbs: 36 g

Fiber: 0 g

Sugar: 0 g

Protein: 6 g

Phosphorus 156 mg

Potassium 231 mg

15. Raspberry Peach Smoothie

Preparation Time: 5 minutes

Cooking Time: 5 minutes

Servings: 1

Ingredients:

- 1 medium peach, sliced
- 1 cup frozen raspberries
- 1 tablespoon honey
- 1/2 cup tofu
- 1 cup unfortified almond milk

Directions:

1. Mix all the ingredients in your blender.

2. Enjoy!

Nutrition:
Protein - 6.3g;

Phosphorus: 29mg;

Potassium: 67mg;

Sodium: 30mg;

Carbs - 23g;

Fat - 3.2g;

Calories – 129.

16. Edamame Guacamole

Preparation Time: 10 minutes

Cooking Time: 0 minute

Servings: 4

Ingredients:

- 1 cup frozen shelled edamame, thawed
- 1/4 cup water
- Juice and zest of 1 lemon
- 2 tablespoons chopped fresh cilantro
- 1 tablespoon olive oil
- 1 teaspoon minced garlic

Directions:

1. In a food processor (or blender), add the edamame, water, lemon juice, lemon zest, cilantro, olive oil, and garlic, and pulse until blended but still a bit chunky.

2. Serve fresh.

Nutrition:

Calories: 63 kcal

Total Fat: 5 g

Saturated Fat: 0 g

Cholesterol: 2 mg

Sodium: 3 mg

Total Carbs: 1 g

Fiber: 0 g

Sugar: 0 g

Protein: 3 g

Phosphorus

Potassium

17. Ginger Cauliflower Rice

Preparation Time: 10 minutes

Cooking Time: 10 minutes

Servings: 4

Ingredients:

- 5 cups cauliflower florets
- 3 tablespoons coconut oil
- 4 ginger slices, grated
- 1 tablespoon coconut vinegar
- 3 garlic cloves, minced
- 1 tablespoon chives, minced
- A pinch of sea salt
- Black pepper to taste

Directions:

1. Put cauliflower florets in a food processor and pulse well.
2. Heat up a pan with the oil over medium-high heat, add ginger, stir and cook for 3 minutes.
3. Add cauliflower rice and garlic, stir and cook for 7 minutes.
4. Add salt, black pepper, vinegar, and chives, stir, cook for a few seconds more, divide between plates and serve.
5. Enjoy!

Nutrition:

Calories 125,

Fat 10, 4,

Fiber 3, 2,

Carbs 7, 9,

Protein 2, 7

Phosphorus: 110mg

Potassium: 117mg

Sodium: 75mg

18. Basil Zucchini Spaghetti

Preparation Time: 1 hour and 10 minutes

Cooking Time: 10 minutes

Servings: 4

Ingredients:

- 1/3 cup coconut oil, melted
- 4 zucchinis, cut with a spiralizer
- 1/4 cup basil, chopped
- A pinch of sea salt
- Black pepper to taste
- 1/2 cup walnuts, chopped
- 2 garlic cloves, minced

Directions:

1. In a bowl, mix zucchini spaghetti with salt and pepper, toss to coat, leave aside for 1 hour, drain well and put in a bowl.
2. Heat up a pan with the oil over medium-high heat, add zucchini spaghetti and garlic, stir and cook for 5 minutes.
3. Add basil and walnuts and black pepper, stir and cook for 3 minutes more.
4. Divide between plates and serve as a side dish
5. Enjoy!

Nutrition:

Calories 287,

Fat 27, 8,

Fiber 3, 3,

Carbs 8, 7,

Protein 6, 3

Phosphorus: 110mg

Potassium: 117mg

Sodium: 75mg

19. Braised Cabbage

Preparation Time: 10 minutes

Cooking Time: 10 minutes

Servings: 4

Ingredients:

- 1 small cabbage head, shredded
- 2 tablespoons water
- A drizzle of olive oil
- 6 ounces shallots, cooked and chopped
- A pinch of black pepper
- A pinch of sweet paprika
- 1 tablespoon dill, chopped

Directions:

1. Heat up a pan with the oil over medium heat, add the cabbage and the water, stir and sauté for 5 minutes.
2. Add the rest of the ingredients, toss, cook for 5 minutes more, divide everything between plates and serve as a side dish!
3. Enjoy!

Nutrition:

Calories 91,

Fat 0, 5,

Fiber 5, 8,

Carbs 20, 8,

Protein 4, 1

Phosphorus: 120mg

Potassium: 127mg

Sodium: 75mg

20. Cauliflower and Leeks

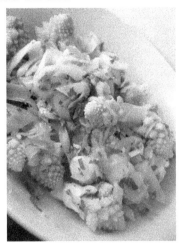

Preparation Time: 10 minutes

Cooking Time: 20 minutes

Servings: 4

Ingredients:

- 1 and 1/2 cups leeks, chopped
- 1 and 1/2 cups cauliflower florets
- 2 garlic cloves, minced
- 1 and 1/2 cups artichoke hearts
- 2 tablespoons coconut oil, melted
- Black pepper to taste

Directions:

1. Heat up a pan with the oil over medium-high heat, add garlic, leeks, cauliflower florets and artichoke hearts, stir and cook for 20 minutes.
2. Add black pepper, stir, divide between plates and serve.
3. Enjoy!

Nutrition:

Calories 192,

Fat 6, 9,

Fiber 8, 2,

Carbs 35, 1,

Protein 5, 1

Phosphorus: 110mg

Potassium: 117mg

Sodium: 75mg

21. Eggplant and Mushroom Sauté

Preparation Time: 10 minutes

Cooking Time: 30 minutes

Servings: 4

Ingredients:

- 2 pounds oyster mushrooms, chopped
- 6 ounces shallots, peeled, chopped
- 1 yellow onion, chopped
- 2 eggplants, cubed
- 3 celery stalks, chopped
- 1 tablespoon parsley, chopped
- A pinch of sea salt
- Black pepper to taste
- 1 tablespoon savory, dried
- 3 tablespoons coconut oil, melted

Directions:

1. Heat up a pan with the oil over medium high heat, add onion, stir and cook for 4 minutes.
2. Add shallots, stir and cook for 4 more minutes.
3. Add eggplant pieces, mushrooms, celery, savory and black pepper to taste, stir and cook for 15 minutes.
4. Add parsley, stir again, cook for a couple more minutes, divide between plates and serve.
5. Enjoy!

Nutrition:

Calories 1013,

Fat 10, 9,

Fiber 35, 5,

Carbs 156, 5,

Protein 69, 1

Phosphorus: 210mg

Potassium: 217mg

Sodium: 105mg

22. Mint Zucchini

Preparation Time: 10 minutes

Cooking Time: 7 minutes

Servings: 4

Ingredients:

- 2 tablespoons mint
- 2 zucchinis, halved lengthwise and then slice into half moons
- 1 tablespoon coconut oil, melted
- 1/2 tablespoon dill, chopped
- A pinch of cayenne pepper

Directions:

1. Heat up a pan with the oil over medium-high heat, add zucchinis, stir and cook for 6 minutes.
2. Add cayenne, dill and mint, stir, cook for 1 minute more, divide between plates and serve.
3. Enjoy!

Nutrition:

Calories 46,

Fat 3, 6,

Fiber 1, 3,

Carbs 3, 5,

Protein 1, 3

Phosphorus: 120mg

Potassium: 127mg

Sodium: 75mg

23. Celery and Kale Mix

Preparation Time: 10 minutes

Cooking Time: 20 minutes

Servings: 4

Ingredients:

- 2 celery stalks, chopped
- 5 cups kale, torn
- 1 small red bell pepper, chopped
- 3 tablespoons water
- 1 tablespoon coconut oil, melted

Directions:

1. Heat up a pan with the oil over medium-high heat, add celery, stir and cook for 10 minutes.
2. Add kale, water, and bell pepper, stir and cook for 10 minutes more.
3. Divide between plates and serve.
4. Enjoy!

Nutrition:

Calories 81,

Fat 3, 5,

Fiber 1, 8,

Carbs 11, 3,

Protein 2, 9

Phosphorus: 120mg

Potassium: 147mg

Sodium: 75mg

24. Kale, Mushrooms and Red Chard Mix

Preparation Time: 10 minutes

Cooking Time: 17 minutes

Servings: 4

Ingredients:

- 1/2 pound brown mushrooms, sliced
- 5 cups kale, roughly chopped
- 1 and 1/2 tablespoons coconut oil
- 3 cups red chard, chopped
- 2 tablespoons water
- Black pepper to taste

Directions:

1. Heat up a pan with the oil over medium high heat, add mushrooms, stir and cook for 5 minutes.
2. Add red chard, kale and water, stir and cook for 10 minutes.
3. Add black pepper to taste, stir and cook 2 minutes more.
4. Divide between plates and serve.
5. Enjoy!

Nutrition:

Calories 97,

Fat 3, 4,

Fiber 2, 3,

Carbs 13, 3,

Protein 5, 4

Phosphorus: 110mg

Potassium: 117mg

Sodium: 75mg

25. Bok Choy and Beets

Preparation Time: 10 minutes

Cooking Time: 30 minutes

Servings: 4

Ingredients:

- 1 tablespoon coconut oil
- 4 cups bok choy, chopped
- 3 beets, cut into quarters and thinly sliced
- 2 tablespoons water
- A pinch of cayenne pepper

Directions:

1. Put water in a large saucepan, add the beets, bring to a boil over medium heat, cover, and cook for 20 minutes and drain.
2. Heat up a pan with the oil over medium high heat, add the bok choy and the water, stir and cook for 10 minutes.
3. Add beets and cayenne pepper, stir, cook for 2 minutes more, divide between plates and serve as a side dish!
4. Enjoy!

Nutrition:

Calories 71,

Fat 3, 7,

Fiber 2, 2,

Carbs 9,

Protein 2, 3

Phosphorus: 110mg

Potassium: 117mg

Sodium: 75mg

26. Spicy Sweet Potatoes

Preparation Time: 10 minutes

Cooking Time: 40 minutes

Servings: 4

Ingredients:

- 4 sweet potatoes, peeled and thinly sliced
- 2 teaspoons nutmeg, ground
- 2 tablespoon coconut oil, melted
- Cayenne pepper to taste

Directions:

1. In a bowl, mix sweet potato slices with nutmeg, cayenne, and oil and toss to coat well.
2. Spread these on a lined baking sheet, place in the oven at 350 degrees F and bake for 25 minutes.
3. Flip the potatoes, bake for 15 minutes more, divide between plates and serve as a side dish.
4. Enjoy!

Nutrition:

Calories 242,

Fat 7, 5,

Fiber 6, 4,

Carbs 42, 4,

Protein 2, 4

Phosphorus: 120mg

Potassium: 137mg

Sodium: 75mg

27. Broccoli and Almonds Mix

Preparation Time: 10 minutes

Cooking Time: 11 minutes

Servings: 4

Ingredients:

- 1 tablespoon olive oil
- 1 garlic clove, minced
- 1 pound broccoli florets
- 1/3 cup almonds, chopped
- Black pepper to taste

Directions:

1. Heat up a pan with the oil over medium-high heat, add the almonds, stir, cook for 5 minutes and transfer to a bowl,
2. Heat up the same pan again over medium-high heat, add broccoli and garlic, stir, cover and cook for 6 minutes more.
3. Add the almonds and black pepper to taste, stir, divide between plates and serve.
4. Enjoy!

Nutrition:

Calories 116,

Fat 7, 8,

Fiber 4,

Carbs 9, 5,

Protein 4, 9

Phosphorus: 110mg

Potassium: 117mg

Sodium: 75mg

28. Squash and Cranberries

Preparation Time: 10 minutes

Cooking Time: 30 minutes

Servings: 2

Ingredients:

- 1 tablespoon coconut oil
- 1 butternut squash, peeled and cubed
- 2 garlic cloves, minced
- 1 small yellow onion, chopped
- 12 ounces coconut milk
- 1 teaspoon curry powder
- 1 teaspoon cinnamon powder
- 1/2 cup cranberries

Directions:

1. Spread squash pieces on a lined baking sheet, place in the oven at 425 degrees F, bake for 15 minutes and leave to one side.
2. Heat up a pan with the oil over medium high heat, add garlic and onion, stir and cook for 5 minutes.
3. Add roasted squash, stir and cook for 3 minutes.
4. Add coconut milk, cranberries, cinnamon and curry powder, stir and cook for 5 minutes more.
5. Divide between plates and serve as a side dish!
6. Enjoy!

Nutrition:

Calories 518,

Fat 47, 6,

Fiber 7, 3,

Carbs 24, 9,

Protein 5, 3

Phosphorus: 110mg

Potassium: 117mg

Sodium: 75mg

29. Roasted Wedges of Cabbage

Preparation Time: 12 minutes

Cooking Time: 35 minutes

Servings: 2

Ingredients:

- 2 teaspoon sugar
- 1 green cabbage, cut into 1-inch wedges
- 1 tablespoon balsamic vinegar
- 1/4 teaspoon freshly ground pepper
- 2 tablespoon olive oil

Directions:

1. Heat up an oven to 450°F, with baking pan heating inside.

2. Combine sugar and pepper in a small bowl.

3. Brush cabbage wedges with oil. Sprinkle with pepper and sugar.

4. Put the seasoned wedges on the hot baking sheet. Roast until cabbage is browned and tender for 25 minutes.

5. Drizzle with balsamic vinegar.

Nutrition:

Protein - 0.74g;

Phosphorus: 36mg;

Potassium: 194mg;

Sodium: 31mg;

Carbs - 4.0g;

Fat - 1.8g;

Calories - 32.3.

30. Creamy Chard

Preparation Time: 10 minutes

Cooking Time: 10 minutes

Servings: 2

Ingredients:

- Juice of 1/2 lemon
- 1 tablespoon coconut oil
- 12 ounces coconut milk
- 1 bunch chard
- A pinch of sea salt
- Black pepper to taste

Directions:

1. Heat up a pan with the oil over medium-high heat, add chard, stir and cook for 5 minutes.
2. Add lemon juice, a pinch of salt, black pepper, and coconut milk, stir and cook for 5 minutes more.
3. Divide between plates and serve as a side.
4. Enjoy!

Nutrition:

Calories 453,

Fat 47, 4,

Fiber 4,

Carbs 10, 1,

Protein 4, 2

Phosphorus: 130mg

Potassium: 1127mg

Sodium: 85mg

31. Dill Carrots

Preparation Time: 10 minutes

Cooking Time: 30 minutes

Servings: 4

Ingredients:

- 1 tablespoon coconut oil, melted
- 2 tablespoons dill, chopped
- 1 pound baby carrots
- 1 tablespoon coconut sugar
- A pinch of black pepper

Directions:

1. Put carrots in a large saucepan, add water to cover, bring to a boil over medium-high heat, cover and simmer for 30 minutes.
2. Drain the carrots, put them in a bowl, add melted oil, black pepper, dill, and the coconut sugar, stir very well, divide between plates and serve.
3. Enjoy!

Nutrition:

Calories 85,

Fat 3, 6,

Fiber 3, 5,

Carbs 13, 4,

Protein 1

Phosphorus: 140mg

Potassium: 147mg

Sodium: 65mg

32. Savory Collard Chips

Preparation Time: 5 minutes

Cooking Time: 20 minutes

Servings: 4

Ingredients:

- 1 bunch of collard greens
- 1 teaspoon of extra-virgin olive oil
- Juice of 1/2 lemon
- 1/2 teaspoon of garlic powder
- 1/4 teaspoon of freshly ground black pepper

Directions:

1. Heat an oven to 350°F. Line a baking sheet with parchment paper.
2. Cut the collards into 2-by-2-inch squares and pat dry with paper towels.
3. Toss greens with the olive oil, lemon juice, garlic powder, and pepper in a large bowl. Use your hands to mix well, massaging the dressing into the greens until evenly coated.
4. Arrange the collards in a single layer on the baking sheet, and cook for 8 minutes. Flip the pieces and cook for an additional 8 minutes, until crisp. Remove from oven, let cool.

Nutrition:

Calories: 24

Total Fat: 1g

Saturated Fat: 0g

Cholesterol: 0mg

Carbs: 3g

Fiber: 1g

Protein: 1g

Phosphorus: 6mg

Potassium: 72mg

Sodium: 8mg

33. Roasted Red Pepper Hummus

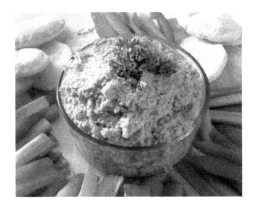

Preparation Time: 10 minutes

Cooking Time: 10 minutes

Servings: 8

Ingredients:

- 1 red bell pepper
- 1 (15-ounce) can of chickpeas, drained and rinsed
- Juice of 1 lemon
- 2 tablespoons of tahini
- 2 garlic cloves
- 2 tablespoons of extra-virgin olive oil

Directions:

1. Move the rack of the oven to the highest position. Heat the broiler to high.

2. Core the pepper and cut it into three or four large pieces. Arrange them on a baking sheet, skin-side up.

3. Broil the peppers for 5 to 10 minutes, until the skins are charred. Remove from the oven then transfer the peppers to a small bowl. Cover with plastic wrap and let them steam for 10 to 15 minutes, until cool enough to handle.

4. Peel the charred skin off the peppers, and place the peppers in a blender.

5. Add the chickpeas, lemon juice, tahini, garlic, and olive oil. Wait until smooth, then add up to 1 tablespoon of water to adjust consistency as desired.

Nutrition:

Calories: 103

Total Fat: 6g

Saturated Fat: 1g

Cholesterol: 0mg

Carbs: 10g

Fiber: 3g

Protein: 3g

Phosphorus: 58mg

Potassium: 91mg

Sodium: 72mg

34. Thai-Style Eggplant Dip

Preparation Time: 10 minutes

Cooking Time: 30 minutes

Servings: 4

Ingredients:

- 1 pound of Thai eggplant (or Japanese or Chinese eggplant)
- 2 tablespoons of rice vinegar
- 2 teaspoons of sugar
- 1 teaspoon of low-sodium soy sauce
- 1 jalapeño pepper
- 2 garlic cloves
- 1/4 cup of chopped basil
- Cut vegetables or crackers, for serving

Directions:

1. Heat an oven to 425°F to get it ready.

2. Pierce every eggplant with a skewer or knife. Place on a rimmed baking sheet and cook until soft, about 30 minutes. Let cool, cut in half, and scoop out the flesh of the eggplant into a blender.

3. Add the rice vinegar, sugar, soy sauce, jalapeño, garlic, and basil to the blender. Process until smooth. Serve with cut vegetables or crackers.

Nutrition:

Calories: 40

Total Fat: 0g

Saturated Fat: 0g

Cholesterol: 0mg

Carbs: 10g

Fiber: 4g

Protein: 2g

Phosphorus: 34mg

Potassium: 284mg

Sodium: 47mg

35. Coconut Pancakes

Preparation Time: 5 minutes

Cooking Time: 10 minutes

Servings: 2

Ingredients:

- 2 free-range egg whites
- 2 tbsp. of all-purpose white flour
- 3 tbsp. of coconut shavings
- 2 tbsp. of coconut milk (optional)
- 1 tbsp. of coconut oil

Directions:

1. Get a bowl and combine all the ingredients.

2. Mix well until you get a thick batter.

3. Heat a skillet on medium heat and heat the coconut oil.

4. Pour half the mixture to the center of the pan, forming a pancake and cook through for 3-4 minutes on each side.

5. Serve with your choice of berries on the top.

Nutrition:

Calories: 177

Fat: 13g

Carbs: 12g

Phosphorus: 37mg

Potassium: 133mg

Sodium: 133mg

Protein: 5g

36. Spiced Peaches

Preparation Time: 5 minutes

Cooking Time: 10 minutes

Servings: 2

Ingredients:

- 1 cup of canned peaches in their own juices
- 1/2 tsp. of cornstarch
- 1 tsp. of ground cloves
- 1 tsp. of ground cinnamon
- 1 tsp. of ground nutmeg
- 1/2 lemon zest
- 1/2 cup of water

Directions:

1. Drain peaches.

2. Combine water, cornstarch, cinnamon, nutmeg, ground cloves, and lemon zest in a pan on the stove.

3. Heat on medium heat and add peaches.

4. Bring to a boil, reduce the heat and simmer for 10 minutes.

5. Serve warm.

Nutrition:

Calories: 70

Fat: 1g

Carbs: 18g

Phosphorus: 26mg

Potassium: 184mg

Sodium: 9mg

Protein: 1g

37. Blueberry and Vanilla Mini Muffins

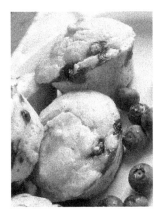

Preparation Time: 10 minutes

Cooking Time: 35 minutes

Servings: 5

Ingredients:

- 3 egg whites
- 1/4 cup of all-purpose white flour
- 1 tbsp. of coconut flour
- 1 tsp. of baking soda
- 1 tbsp. of nutmeg, grated
- 1 tsp. of vanilla extract
- 1 tsp. of stevia
- 1/4 cup of fresh blueberries

Directions:

1. Set the oven 325°F/170°C/Gas Mark 3 for Preheating.

2. Add all the ingredients in a bowl.

3. Divide the batter into 4 and spoon into a lightly oiled muffin tin.

4. Bake in the oven for 15–20 minutes or until cooked through.

5. Your knife should pull out clean from the middle of the muffin once done.

6. Allow to cool on a wired rack before serving.

Nutrition:

Calories: 48

Fat: 1g

Carbs: 8g

Phosphorus: 14mg

Potassium: 44mg

Sodium: 298mg

Protein: 2g

38. Puffy French toast

Preparation Time: 10 minutes

Cooking Time: 8 minutes

Servings: 4

Ingredients:

- 4 slices of white bread, cut in half diagonally
- 3 whole eggs and 1 egg white
- 1 cup of plain almond milk
- 2 tbsp. of canola oil
- 1 tsp. of cinnamon

Directions:

1. Preheat your oven to 400F/180C

2. Beat the eggs and the almond milk.

3. Heat the oil in a pan.

4. Dip each bread slice/triangle into the egg and almond milk mixture.

5. Fry in the pan until golden brown on each side.

6. Place the toasts in a baking sheet and let cook in the oven for another 5 minutes.

7. Serve warm and drizzle with some honey, icing sugar, or cinnamon on top.

Nutrition:

Calories: 293.75

Carbs: 25.3g

Protein: 9.27g

Sodium: 211g

Potassium: 97mg

Phosphorus: 165mg

Dietary Fiber: 12.3g

Fat: 16.50g

39. Puff Oven Pancakes

Preparation Time: 5 minutes

Cooking Time: 30 minutes

Servings: 4

Ingredients:

- 2 large eggs.
- 1/2 cup of rice flour
- 1/2 cup of rice milk
- 2 tbsp. of unsalted butter
- 1/8 tsp. of salt

Directions:

1. Preheat the oven at 400°F/190°C.

2. Grease a 10-inch skillet or Pyrex with the butter and heat in the oven until it melts.

3. Beat the eggs and whisk in the rice milk, flour and salt in a mixing bowl until smooth.

4. Take off the skillet or pie dish from the oven.

5. Transfer the batter directly into the skillet and put back in the oven for 25–30 minutes.

6. Place in a serving dish and cut into 4 portions.

7. Serve hot with honey or icing sugar on top.

Nutrition:

Calories: 159.75

Fat: 7.18 g

Carbs: 17g

Protein: 5g

Sodium: 120g

Potassium: 52mg

Phosphorus: 66.25mg

40. Savory Muffins with Protein

Preparation Time: 5 minutes

Cooking Time: 35 minutes

Servings: 12

Ingredients:

- 2 cups of corn flakes
- 1/2 cup of unfortified almond milk
- 4 large eggs
- 2 tbsp. of olive oil
- 1/2 cup of almond milk
- 1 medium white onion, sliced
- 1 cup of plain Greek yogurt
- 1/4 cup of pecans, chopped
- 1 tbsp. of mixed seasoning blend, e.g., Mrs. dash

Directions:

1. Preheat the oven at 350°F/180°C.

2. Heat the olive oil in the pan. Sauté the onions with the pecans and seasoning blend for a couple of minutes.

3. Add the rest of the ingredients and toss well.

4. Split the mixture into 12 small muffin cups (lightly greased) and bake for 30–35 minutes or until an inserted knife or toothpick is coming out clean.

5. Serve warm or keep at room temperature for a couple of days.

Nutrition:

Calories: 106.58

Fat: 6.8 g

Carbs: 8.20g

Protein: 4.77g

Sodium: 51.91mg

Potassium: 87.83 mg

Phosphorus: 49.41 mg

41. European Pancakes

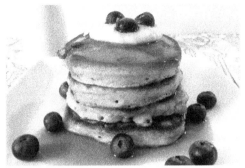

Preparation Time: 5 minutes

Cooking Time: 20 minutes

Servings: 10

Ingredients:

- 2/3 cups of all-purpose flour
- 4 large eggs
- 2 tbsp. of sugar
- 1/2 tsp. of lemon zest
- 1 cup of low-Fat milk
- 1/4 tsp. of vanilla extract

Directions:

1. Mix flour and sugar, then whisk in the eggs and combine well in a medium.

2. Put then the milk, vanilla, and lemon zest to the mix and whisk well.

3. Spray a small 8–10-inch pan with cooking spray and pour around 4 tbsp. of the mixture and distribute evenly by tilting the pan from one side to another.

4. Cook until the batter is solid and light golden brown (around 50 seconds on each side). Flip.

5. Repeat the above two steps until all the batter has finished.

Nutrition:

Calories: 74

Carbs: 10g

Protein: 4g

Sodium: 39mg

Potassium: 73mg

Phosphorus: 73mg

42. Easy and Fast Mac-n-Cheese

Preparation Time: 5 minutes

Cooking Time: 8-10 minutes

Servings: 4

Ingredients:

- 1 cup of dry elbow macaroni pasta
- 1/2 cup of mild cheddar cheese
- 3 cups of water
- 1 tsp. of unsalted butter
- 1/2 tsp. of dry mustard powder
- 1/2 tsp. of paprika

Directions:

1. Boil the elbow macaroni in boiling water for 7–8 minutes (or until soft).

2. Drain all the water out and transfer it in the bowl.

3. Add the butter cheese, mustard, and paprika while the pasta is still hot, toss and serve.

Nutrition:

Calories: 231.68

Fat: 1.1 g

Carbs: 32.65g

Protein: 9.74g

Sodium: 107.25mg

Potassium: 29.52mg

Phosphorus: 159.93mg

43. Sandwich with Chicken Salad

Preparation Time: 10 minutes

Cooking Time: 10 minutes

Servings: 2

Ingredients:

- 2 bowls of cooked chicken
- 1/2 cup of low-Fat mayonnaise
- 1/2 cup of green bell pepper
- 1 cup of pieces pineapple
- 1/3 cup of carrots
- 4 slices of flatbread
- 1/2 tsp. of black pepper

Directions:

1. Prepare aside the diced chicken and drain pineapple, adding green bell pepper, black pepper, and carrots.

2. Combine all in a bowl and refrigerate until chilled.

3. Later on, serve the chicken salad on the flatbread. Enjoy!

Nutrition:

Calories: 345

Fat 31.71 g

Protein: 22g

Carbs 105.93 g

Sodium: 395mg

Potassium: 330mg

Phosphorus: 165mg

44. Celery and Arugula Salad

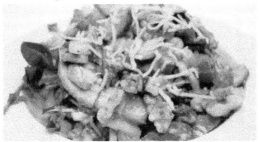

Preparation Time: 10 minutes

Cooking Time: 0 minute

Servings: 4

Ingredients:

- 1 shallot, thinly sliced
- 3 celery stalks, cut into 1-inch pieces about 1/4 inch thick
- 2 cups of loosely packed arugula
- 1 tablespoon of extra-virgin olive oil
- 2 tablespoons of white wine vinegar
- Freshly ground black pepper
- 2 tablespoons of grated Parmesan cheese

Directions:

1. In a medium bowl, toss the shallot, celery stalks, and arugula.

2. In a small bowl, whisk the olive oil, vinegar, and pepper.

3. Toss your salad with your dressing.

4. Top with Parmesan cheese and serve.

Nutrition:

Calories: 45

Fat: 4g

Carbs: 1g

Protein: 1g

Phosphorus: 23mg

Potassium: 47mg

Sodium: 47mg

45. Crunchy Potato Croquettes

Preparation Time: 15 minutes

Cooking Time: 20 minutes

Servings: 4

Ingredients:

- 4 medium "leached" potato, cooked and peeled
- 1 tbsp. of butter
- 1 tbsp. of rice milk
- 1 tsp. of pepper
- 1 beaten egg
- 1 cup of white bread crumbs
- 2 tbsp. of canola oil

Directions:

1. Mash potatoes with milk, butter, and pepper.

2. Form cooled potatoes into balls with your hands.

3. Dip balls in beaten egg.

4. Next, roll balls in bread crumbs.

5. Then place balls in a hot oiled skillet and fry until golden brown.

Nutrition:

Calories: 322.1

Fat 12.77 g

Carbs 39.06 g

Protein: 7.5g

Sodium: 399.7mg

Phosphorus: 13.5mg

Potassium: 233.5mg

46. Vegetarian Summer Rolls

Preparation Time: 3. Minutes

Cooking Time: 0 minute

Servings: 24

Ingredients:

- 1 ounce of rice vermicelli noodles
- 2 zucchinis shredded
- 2 carrots shredded
- 2 shallots finely chopped
- 2 small cucumbers peeled and diced
- 1/3 cup of fresh basil chopped
- 1/2 cup of fresh cilantro chopped
- 24 spring roll wrappers

Dipping Sauce:

- 1/4 cup of sugar
- 1/4 cup of rice vinegar
- 2 fresh red chilies

Directions:

1. Place sugar, vinegar, and 2 tbsp. of water in a saucepan and boil gently.

2. Remove from heat, add chilies, and set aside.

3. In a large bowl, combine all rest of the ingredients (except wrappers).

4. Place a moistened wrapper on a work surface.

5. Put a spoonful of filling in the center and fold to encase, bringing corner to corner.

6. Fold in sides and roll up tightly. Brush end with water to seal.

7. Repeat until all filling is used.

8. Serve with dipping sauce.

Nutrition:

Calories: 94.5

Fat 0.53 g

Carbs 19.43 g

Protein: 0.2g

Sodium: 562.6mg

Phosphorus: 0.5mg

Potassium 63 mg

47. Strawberry Papaya Smoothie

Preparation Time: 10 minutes

Cooking Time: 0 minutes

Servings: 1

Ingredients:

- 1/2 cup of strawberries
- 2 cups of sliced papaya
- 2 cup of coconut kefir
- 2 scoop of vanilla bone broth Protein powder
- 1/2 cup of ice water

Directions:

1. Add all of the ingredients to the blender and mix until the Strawberry Papaya Smoothie is pleasantly joined. I love including a crisp sprig of mint to supplement this new and fruity smoothie.

Nutrition:

Calories: 105;

Fat: 19g;

Phosphorus: 23mg;

Potassium: 92mg;

Sodium: 24mg;

Carbs: 5g;

Protein: 2.8g.

48. Cinnamon Egg Smoothie

Preparation Time: 10 minutes

Cooking Time: 0 minutes

Servings: 1

Ingredients:

- 1/2 teaspoon ground cinnamon
- 1 teaspoon stevia
- 1/8 teaspoon vanilla extract
- 8 oz. egg white, pasteurized
- 3 tablespoons whipped topping

Directions:

2. Mix the stevia, egg whites, cinnamon, and vanilla in a mixer.

3. Serve with whipped topping.

4. Enjoy.

Nutrition:

Calories 95;

Total Fat 1.2g;

Saturated Fat 0.6g;

Cholesterol 3mg;

Sodium 120mg;

Carbs 3.1g;

Dietary Fiber 0.3g;

Sugars 0.8g;

Protein 12.5g;

Calcium 18mg;

Phosphorus 185mg;

Potassium 194mg.

49. Vanilla Fruit Smoothie

Preparation Time: 10 minutes

Cooking Time: 0 minutes

Servings: 2

Ingredients:

- 2 oz. mango, peeled and cubed
- 2 oz. strawberries
- 2 oz. avocado flesh, cubed
- 2 oz. banana, peeled
- 2 scoops of Protein powder
- 1 cup cold water
- 1 cup crushed ice

Directions:

1. First, begin by putting everything into a blender jug.

2. Pulse it for 30 seconds until well blended.

3. Serve chilled.

Nutrition:

Calories 228;

Total Fat 7.6g;

Saturated Fat 2.1g;

Cholesterol 65mg;

Sodium 58mg;

Total Carbs 19g;

Dietary Fiber 3.6g;

Sugars 9.8g;

Protein 23.4g;

Calcium 112mg;

Phosphorus 216 mg;

Potassium 504mg.

50. Pina Colada Spicy Smoothie

Preparation Time: 2 minutes

Cooking Time: 5 minutes

Servings: 2

Ingredients:

- 1 cup Mascarpone Cheese, firm
- 1 cup pineapple, canned or fresh
- 1 teaspoon Stevia or another sweetener
- 1/2 cup pineapple juice, unsweetened
- Pinch red pepper flakes

Directions:

1. Mix all the ingredients in a blender.

2. Serve.

Nutrition:

Protein - 13.4g;

Phosphorus: 23mg;

Potassium: 55mg;

Sodium: 18mg;

Carbs - 32g;

Fat - 5g;

Calories – 189.

Conclusion

Managing chronic kidney disease (CKD) requires lifestyle adjustments, but it might help to know that you're not alone. Over 31 m. Individuals in the United States are detected with malfunctions of their kidneys or are battling kidney disease. I have helped many people manage the physical symptoms associated with this disease and cope with the emotional toll that this life change can take. Without knowing what the future holds, uncertainty, fear, depression, and anxiety can be common. It may even feel like dialysis is inevitable, and you may be asking yourself if it is worth the time or effort to try and manage this stage of the disease, or if it's even possible to delay the progression. As an expert in this field, I can assure you it is not just possible, it's yours to achieve—only 1 in 50 diagnosed with CKD end up on dialysis. So together, with the right tools, we can work to delay and ultimately prevent end-stage renal disease and dialysis. Success is earned through diet modifications and lifestyle changes. Using simple, manageable strategies, I have watched firsthand as my patients empowered themselves with knowledge. They have gone on to lead full, productive, and happy lives, continuing to work, play, and enjoy spending time with their loved ones—just the way it should be!

Only 1 in 50 diagnosed with CKD end up on dialysis

Diet is a vital part of treatment for CKD, and it can help immensely in slowing the progression of the disease. Some ingredients help the kidneys function, while others make the kidneys work harder. This book has focused on crowding out the unhealthy with healthy and helpful. Also, targeting factors like salt and carbohydrate intake are important to reduce the risk of hypertension, diabetes, and other diseases that can result from kidney failure. I can't emphasize enough the importance of consulting a dietitian throughout CKD progression to optimize health. This book is a good start, as it is designed specifically for the treatment of this population.

In this time of change and uncertainty, the knowledge you gain from these pages will give you the power to take your life into your hands and make changes to benefit you in the short and long term. I hope to educate & inspire you with new, easy ways to change your health trajectory. Adopting a kidney-friendly lifestyle can be challenging at first but following these recipes will reduce the anxiety associated with selecting smart food options for your everyday life. And lest you worry that your new diet is restrictive or unsustainable, I want to assure you that these recipes are both easy and delicious, and they will give you a realistic, satisfying way to make this lifestyle change. This book will be your guide you at each step of the way. Doing so will help take the stress of meal planning out of the equation and help you focus on the truly important things in life.

Conversion Tables

Volume Equivalents (Liquid)

US STANDARD	US STANDARD (OUNCES)	METRIC (APPROXIMATE)
2 tablespoons	1 fl. oz.	30 mL
1/4 cup	2 fl. oz.	60 mL
1/2 cup	4 fl. oz.	120 mL
1 cup	8 fl. oz.	240 mL
1 1/2 cups	12 fl. oz.	355 mL
2 cups or 1 pint	16 fl. oz.	475 mL
4 cups or 1 quart	32 fl. oz.	1 L
1 gallon	128 fl. oz.	4 L

Volume Equivalents (Dry)

US STANDARD	METRIC (APPROXIMATE)
1/4 teaspoon	1 mL
1/2 teaspoon	2 mL
1 teaspoon	5 mL
1 tablespoon	15 mL
1/4 cup	59 mL
cup	79 mL
1/2 cup	118 mL
1 cup	177 mL

Oven Temperatures

FAHRENHEIT (F)	CELSIUS (C) (APPROXIMATE)
250°F	120 °C
300°F	150°C
325°F	165°C
350°F	180°C
375°F	190°C
400°F	200°C
425°F	220°C
450°F	230°C

Weight Equivalents

US STANDARD	METRIC (APPROXIMATE)
1/2 ounce	15 g
1 ounce	30 g
2 ounces	60 g
4 ounces	115 g
8 ounces	225 g
12 ounces	340 g
16 ounces or 1 pound	455 g

References

American Diabetes Association. "Age, Race, Gender & Family History." February 12, 2014. Accessed June 15, 2015. http://www.diabetes.org/are-you-at-risk/lower-your-risk/nonmodifiables.html.

American Dietetic Association. "Pocket Resource for Nutrition Assessment: 2009 Edition." 2009. Accessed June 16, 2015. http://dpg-storage.s3.amazonaws.com/dhcc/resources/PocketResources/PRNA%202009.pdf.

American Kidney Fund. "Kidney Disease Statistics." Accessed June 14, 2015. http://www.kidneyfund.org/about-us/assets/pdfs/akf-kidneydiseasestatistics-2012.pdf.

American Kidney Fund. "Race/Ethnicity and Kidney Disease." Accessed June 15, 2015. http://www.kidneyfund.org/are-you-at-risk/risk-factors/race-kidney-disease.

Centers for Disease Control and Prevention. "National Chronic Kidney Disease Fact Sheet, 2014." 2014. Accessed June 16, 2015. http://www.cdc.gov/diabetes/pubs/pdf/kidney_factsheet.pdf.

Clinical Journal of the American Society of Nephrology. "Prevalence of Chronic Kidney Disease in US Adults with Undiagnosed Diabetes or Prediabetes." January 8, 2010. Accessed June 14, 2015. http://cjasn.asnjournals.org/content/5/4/673.

DaVita HealthCare Partners. "Phosphorus and Chronic Kidney Disease." Accessed June 18, 2015. http://www.davita.com/kidney-disease/diet-and-nutrition/diet-basics/phosphorus-and-chronic-kidney-disease/e/5306.

DaVita HealthCare Partners. "Potassium and Chronic Kidney Disease." Accessed June 18, 2015. http://www.davita.com/kidney-disease/diet-and-nutrition/diet%20basics/potassium-and-chronic-kidney-disease/e/5308.

Kidney & Urology Foundation of America. "High Blood Pressure and Kidney Disease." August 2005. Accessed June 16, 2015. http://www.kidneyurology.org/Library/Kidney_Health/High_Blood_Pressure_and_Kidney_Disease.php.

Krishnamurthy, V., G. Wei, B. Baird, M. Murtaugh, M. Chonchol, K. Raphael, T. Greene, S. Beddhu. "High Dietary Fiber Intake Is Associated w/ Decreased Inflammation and All-Cause Mortality In Patients with Chronic Kidney Disease." Kidney International, 81 (3: February 2012), 300–6. Doi: 10.1038/ki.2011.355.

National Institute of Diabetes & Digestive & Kidney Diseases. "Kidney Disease of Diabetes." April 2, 2004. Accessed June 15, 2015. http://www.niddk.nih.gov/health-information/health-topics/kidney-disease/kidney-disease-of-diabetes/Pages/facts.aspx.

National Institutes of Health. "Kidney Disease: Early Detection and Treatment." NIH Medline plus 3, number 1 (winter 2008): 9–10. Accessed June 15, 2015. http://www.nlm.nih.gov/medlineplus/magazine/issues/winter08/articles/winter08pg9-10.html.

National Kidney Foundation. "About Chronic Kidney Disease." Accessed July 12, 2015. https://www.kidney.org/kidneydisease/aboutckd.

National Kidney Foundation. "Cholesterol and Chronic Kidney Disease." Accessed June 16, 2015. https://www.kidney.org/atoz/content/cholesterol.

National Kidney Foundation. "How Your Kidneys Work." Accessed June 15, 2015. https://www.kidney.org/kidneydisease/howkidneyswrk.

National Kidney Foundation. "KDOQI Clinical Practice Guidelines & Clinical Practice Recommendations for Diabetes & Chronic Kidney Disease." Accessed June 16, 2015. http://www2.kidney.org/professionals/KDOQI/guideline_diabetes/guide5.htm.

National Kidney Foundation. "Phosphorus and Your CKD Diet." Accessed June 16, 2015. https://www.kidney.org/atoz/content/phosphorus.

National Kidney Foundation. "Sodium and Your CKD Diet: How to Spice up Your Cooking." Accessed June 17, 2015. https://www.kidney.org/atoz/content/sodiumckd.

National Kidney Foundation. "Vitamins and Minerals in Kidney Disease." Accessed June 17, 2015. https://www.kidney.org/atoz/content/vitamineral.

The Renal Association. "CKD Stages." Accessed June 16, 2015. http://www.renal.org/information-resources/the-uk-eckd-guide/ckd-stages#sthash.jWT6jJfH.dpbs.

Renal Health Network. "Are Your Kidneys Okay?" Accessed June 15, 2015. http://www.renalhealthnetwork.com/index.php?page=are-your-kidneys-okay.

US Department of Agriculture. "National Agriculture Library: Macronutrients." Accessed June 16, 2015. http://fnic.nal.usda.gov/food-composition/macronutrients.

US Department of Agriculture. "National Nutrient Database for Standard Reference Release 27." Accessed June 16, 2015. http://ndb.nal.usda.gov.

US National Library of Medicine. "Medline Plus: Chronic Kidney Disease." October 2, 2013. Accessed June 16, 2015. http://www.nlm.nih.gov/medlineplus/ency/article/000471.htm.

Credits